Health Is A Journey, Not A Battle

A Wellness Story

Nasha Shandri, CHC, LMT

DEDICATION

This book is dedicated to my beautiful children Zoe and Jon. Mommy loves you sooooo much! I also dedicate this book to all of the men and women that are still trying to figure out their health.

CONTENTS

ACKNOWLEDGMENTS

Special thanks to my husband Ross, my family and friends who have been so supportive of me in my health and wellness journey. May you all continue to be blessed with the same love, courage, and grace you have shown me in this process.

And thank you to my friend, mentor, and sister Lynita Mitchell-Blackwell for encouraging, guiding, and listening.

1 IT'S A LIFESTYLE

I walked in the bar, noticed the unfamiliar faces, and immediately constructed my hometown "Who Are You" face in response to the eyes sizing me up. Then as I scanned to the left, I actually saw a familiar face. "Chantae!" I cried out in joy, my face dissolving from attitude to gratitude as I recognized my longtime friend.

Chantae and I screamed and gripped one another in a near-death hug. Chantae then pushed me back, looking me up from head to toe. It had been years since we last saw one another, and I was noticeably thinner. "Look at you!" Chantae said in awe. "I guess you really do eat those salads you post on Facebook. I would do it, but...." she trailed off with a sigh and half shrug. Then said, "Well, I guess it works huh." I smiled in answer, and we began to talk. Although I tried to steer the conversation away from weight and toward catching up, Chantae circled back to weight loss.

We talked about several diets, Chantae mentioning how she had success losing weight for a wedding with Atkins. We then moved on to our shared love for the brand 1800 (it is a white liquor, and has less calories than its counterparts). She was surprised, since I am the self-styled "Health Stylist" - who knew I partook in the occasional aparatif? (I really blew her away when I shared a tip about increasing vitamin C to help prevent hangover.)

When I saw that Chantae was really feeling what I was saying, I began talking about the great recipes she could create with carrots and kale, and the joys of shopping at the Farmers Market. She shot me a look of suspicion, and cut me off with a roll of her eyes, and asked the question that almost always comes next: "What's your secret - really?"

The secret is... I don't have a secret, I have a lifestyle. I consistently make small choices to better serve my goal. My goal is not to spend my life in the gym. I would rather spend time with my family, friends, volunteering in the community, and sharing my wellness journey with others. No hate on the gym rats - if that is how you like to spend your time, more power to you, but I have other interests.

Now, don't get me wrong: movement is necessary. We must keep our bodies moving and burning energy to remain healthy. But health is more than working out, and it is more than what we consume. True health is how we LIVE. And my number one trick to living well is so simple, most people will miss it: <u>it's all in the glass</u>.

A glass? Not hours at the gym, or yo-yo dieting, or countless supplements or enough water to make you float away??? Nope, not for me. My key to maintaining double-digit pound weight reduction and 6 dress size loss over 15 years has been my commitment to the super-smoothie.

Now, let's face it. There are TONS of books and programs out there that claim to have the answer for helping you to lose weight, reverse disease, and otherwise reclaim your health. But no one book has every single person's "right" answer. If it did, there would only be one book! That being said, when it comes to achieving optimal health, there are a few basic principles that apply to almost everyone. <u>The most basic universal principle is that we all need to eat more plants:</u> dark, nutrient, dense, leafy greens; vegetables; and fruits of all colors, shapes and sizes. These natural foods hold the key to health and longevity for us all.

I will be the first to admit that it is hard to actually consume enough of these super-foods in quantities that will make a real and noticeable difference in our lives. That is – unless you throw them all in a blender and drink them!

What?

Yes, my secret in a glass is the Green Smoothie.

This is the magic bullet, the piece de resistance, the end all-be all of food health. If there was only one thing you could do for your health that would make an immediate, noticeable difference that would last the rest of your life, drinking this daily is the way to do it. If you can squeeze in a second, that is even better!

Here's another confession: the Green Smoothie is not the prettiest girl at the dance. As a matter of fact, she would be better described as the girl with the great personality who wins you over once you get to know her. Upon first sight, the Green Smoothie kind of looks like rich soil with gummy worms emerging through the surface. Appealing to third graders, but not so much to adults with more, shall we say, refined tastes.

Why is that? I believe it is because the Green Smoothie is.... well... GREEN! Too many of us adults have lost our sense of adventure! If you really want to enjoy healthy living and eating, you have to embrace a sense of daring. It will be rewarded - promise! Once you close your eyes and taste the Green Smoothie, it's like ambrosia. The key is to blend it thoroughly.

When properly blended, the Green Smoothie is a delightfully refreshing treat that transcends the color in the glass. And when you realize all the health benefits of drinking green smoothies, you won't want to live without them.

2 WHY GREENS?

The most nutrient dense foods on the planet are leafy green vegetables. Foods like spinach, kale, collards, swiss chard, bok choy, watercress, parsley, mustard greens, and turnip greens are super charged with nutrients. They also contain the purist form of nutrients with the fewest amount of calories per serving. So if you want to lose weight, eat your greens!

Growing up, I remember my mother admonishing us to eat our veggies. I am in my late thirties now, and the world has changed. Americans now eat fewer leafy green vegetables than any other food. We need these super foods most, yet we eat them least of all. That is a dangerous trend that our collective waistlines prove is destroying our lifestyles and life-spans.

Why won't we eat greens? Part of the reason is because greens are not the easiest foods to eat. I'm not talking about greens found in salads, rather those that require preparation. Effort is required to prepare greens so that they provide the maximum amount of nutrients, taste good, and are easy to chew and swallow.

The way around this seemingly gigantic hurdle is to throw your greens into a blender and create a smoothie! Adding greens to your smoothie is simple and convenient, and when combined with fruits, the taste is hardly noticeable.

3 THE BLENDER IS KING

Blending your Green Smoothie is the best way to get all the benefits of drinking green and sidestep the roadblocks to eating well. Blending is not only a convenient way to get your greens, but also a *superior* way:

1. **Quantity**: To get the most out of eating leafy greens, you need to eat a LOT of them. This is actually a time consuming task, and unless you love greens more than any other food on the planet and plan to eat several large salads a day, you aren't likely to eat them in the quantities that will deliver serious health benefits. I personally find that I am able to consume three times as many greens in a smoothie as I am in a salad or steamed dish.

2. **Taste**: After revealing my Green Smoothie "secret", a friend told me her smoothies tasted too earthy, like dirt. So you may not be ready for the "mean green" smoothie recipe that is full of veggies... and that's okay - give yourself some time. Our modern processed

diet filled with foods containing artificial flavors and sweeteners have compromised our taste buds, making it hard to appreciate the taste of greens. Hiding them in a smoothie is the perfect way to enjoy eating well.

3. **Benefits of Raw**: There is a lot of evidence pointing to the benefits of eating raw foods. Most plants, when cooked, tend to lose their nutrients to varying degrees. Such loss depends on the temperature at which they are cooked and the method (baked versus broiled versus fried versus grilled). Since the greens in your smoothie are always raw, you get the benefit of all the nutrients in their purest, whole food state.

4. **Digestion:** Greens are called roughage for a reason; they can be pretty rough on our intestinal tracts. And when we chew, we don't always get all the benefits of the food. According to Dr. Joel Fuhrman, longtime advocate of achieving nutritional excellence through the consumption of a plant-based diet, "When we simply chew a salad, about 70 to 90 percent of the [plant] cells are not broken open. As a result, most of the valuable nutrients contained within those cells never enter our bloodstream." He considers what he calls a "blended salad" a "powerful and delicious way to maximize your intake of nutrients." Since the food in a smoothie has already been mostly liquefied from going through the blender,

your body will digest the food much more easily, and assimilate the

nutrients much faster. When your body gets the nutrients into

your system, you will immediately feel the difference!

4 MY PERSONAL TIPPING POINT - PART 1

I started making smoothies in 2009 after my son's birth. I was so busy with two small children, a new business, and wifely duties, some days "I didn't know if I was coming or going" as the old folks used to say. One thing I did know: I was not consuming enough nutrients to nurse properly. As a wellness advocate, I knew I had to feed myself and my family properly. I set out to find the most amazing green smoothie recipe, and after many months, I did. It is my pleasure to share it with you, but a few words of caution:

1. If you are diabetic, consult with your doctor before trying these recipes as they contain a large portion of fruit, which is high in sugar.

2. Use the highest quality apple juice and orange juice you can get your hands on.

Okay, here are my recipes for great health:

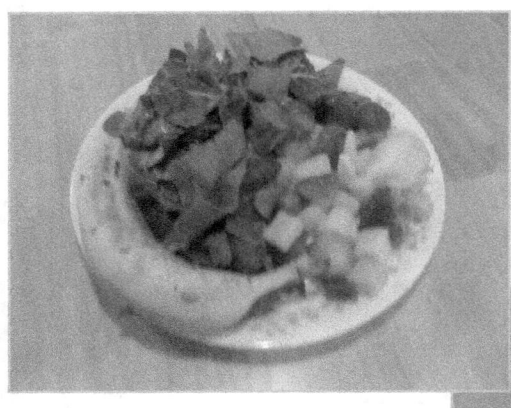

Each photo above represents the amount of food that goes into just ONE 16 oz. green smoothie!

The Basic Three Minute Green Smoothie

You'll need:

- **A blender.** The higher powered, the better. But really, any blender that works will do the trick. Don't delay simply because you don't have a power blender like a Blendtec or Vitamix on your kitchen counter!

- **Up to eight cups of loose, leafy green vegetables.** The amount is purely based on what you want to achieve. If you want to ease into the smoothies and are a bit apprehensive about the taste of them in a blended drink, a handful of spinach is a great place to start. If you want to be amazed by the jolt of energy and clarity you'll feel after drinking one, you'll want to fill your blender (loosely!) to the top with one or more of the variety of greens listed earlier in this chapter.

- **Two or three ripe bananas – if you have insulin/glucose issues substitute with half an avocado for the creamy texture**

- **A 12 or 16 oz bag of frozen fruit** – just be sure there is NOTHING added to the bag besides pure fruit

- **3 cups of pure water** (more or less to taste)

Start by filling your blender with the greens, then add the water and blend thoroughly. If you've filled the blender to the top with the greens, the volume should come down about halfway after blended.

Peel and add the bananas. You may want to start with two and see how full your blender becomes, but if the bananas are small, be sure to add the third for the creamy consistency and natural sweetness necessary to counter the taste of any greens.

Add your bag of fruit. Because the fruit is frozen, the nutrients are just as powerful, if not more so, than in fresh fruit. The convenience of a frozen bag of fruit can't be denied – no peeling, no washing, no mess. And the frozen factor means you don't have to add ice to get the smoothie to be – well, a smoothie!

The first few times you do this, you may find you have to experiment a bit with the amounts of water and greens that feel right to you. So give yourself a bit of time.

> *The key to the smoothie is blending it well, so that no lumps prevent you from enjoying it.*

Adding Other Ingredients

This is the basic, simple, straightforward, nutrient powerhouse smoothie. While you don't need to add other ingredients, you might want to, for the benefit of taste or nutrition. Looking for more flavor, try an all natural fruit juice. Orange or apple would be simple, but there are lots of exotic options out there too, such as mango, pineapple, or pomegranate. Just stay away from anything that contains added sugar, syrup, or preservatives – just stick to juice.

If you want a more creamy consistency, you might try milk, soy or almond milk, or yogurt. (Beware: dairy products might counteract the effects of the energy in the whole foods, depending on what your body can tolerate. And <u>if you're trying to lose weight, it's best to stick with just water</u>.)

To add layers of nutrition, you can certainly add other fresh fruits and vegetables – any of them will work. One friend of mine loves to add hemp seeds in hers, and one of my clients can't stand the taste of carrots but has figured out how to add them and hide their taste in a smoothie. I've used frozen spinach and broccoli as well – you just need to let the vegetables thaw a bit before subjecting your blender to them.

The possibilities and combinations are endless if you really want to be adventurous. There are lots of resources out there to help you sort through the options.

<u>When and How To Enjoy</u>

If you're one of those people who feels as if you don't have time for a healthy breakfast, well now you do, and research suggests that eating plants first thing in the morning is an extremely healthy way to start your day. It only takes three minutes to whip up this recipe if you want it fresh. You can prepare it the night before and have it ready if you. If you've made a whole pitcher, you might also try filling a portable shaker bottle so you can enjoy one before lunch, for lunch, or as a snack. Just store it in a refrigerator, and leave enough room in the bottle to be able to shake the contents, as they will settle and thicken over the course of a few hours.

This method keeps it simple. But if you'd like to add some spice and variety to your smoothies, allow me to suggest you take the Green Smoothie Challenge: www.greensmoothiechallenge.com.

The above recipes introduced my children and I to kale. I will admit during the winter months I did not have smoothies daily, but the spring rejuvenated my taste buds, so I dove in with gusto. I would venture to coconut water as my liquid and use spinach, swiss chard, and different varieties of lettuce. We played around with the ingredients to manipulate the smoothie colors. We experienced orange, blue, yellow, and... brown. We learned that brown is the result of mixing too many colors. If you are a brown fan, then go all in! But if you are just starting out, you may want to hold back a little so you may enjoy a more colorful experience.

Weight Loss & Maintenance

Smoothies are not the end-all, be-all for maintaining a healthy and consistent size and weight. You still need to practice self control and discipline regarding the other things you eat and drink, and maintain an active lifestyle. However, smoothies can be one of the easiest weight loss kick starters and weight maintenance tools to help on your journey to wellness.

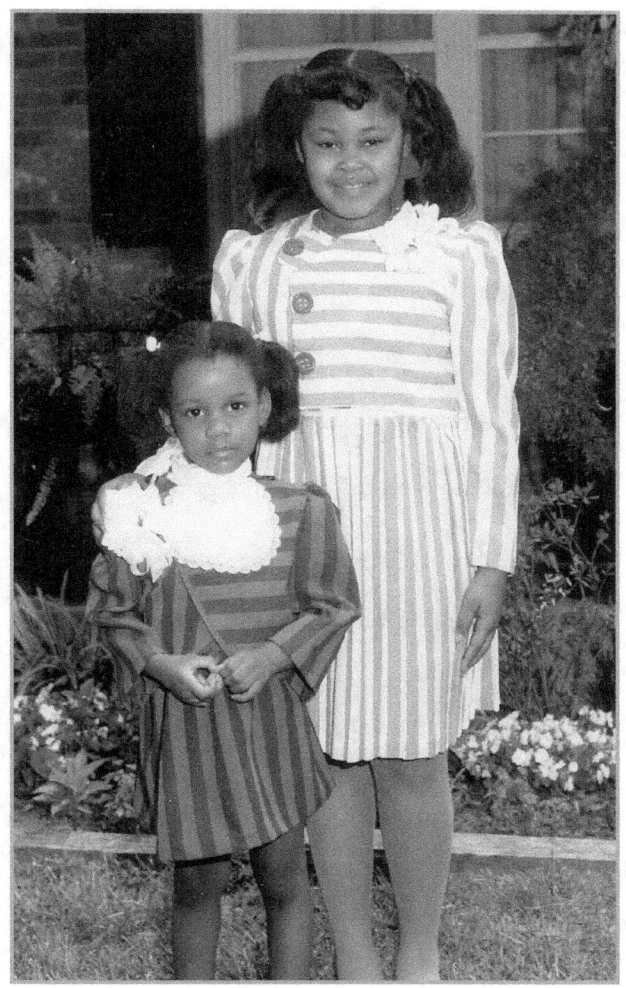

Ten years old, with my younger sister.

My personal story is probably like many of those who have struggled

with their waistlines. Hard to believe it now, but I was a hefty kid growing

up. My family was very loving, my friends were great, and so I never

thought about or noticed my size until the third grade.

I vividly remember being with my classmates at our teacher's house for the end of the year cook out. We were playing red rover. My classmates yelled, "Red rover, red rover, send Nasha right over." I went for the hand-chain that I perceived to be the "weakest link", a place where I could easily break through. I ran to the other side, all smiles into the arms of my two classmates... And broke the chain. I made it through, I'd won! But there was crying and angst behind me. I was so confused. What happened? I had hurt my classmate. Apparently my weight, when added to my speed were too much for the little girl's arm, and I caused her pain when I came through the human chain. Her mother comforted her, but glared at me with a mixture of horror and resentment. I was only eight years old, yet I remember it all as if it were yesterday. The embarrassment, shame, and regret all rolled up in my little heart to carry with me well into adulthood.

Just three years later, my size once again became an issue of fixation in my young life. I was home trying on a new pair of pants in my bedroom when I overhear one of my aunts ask my mom how I had "gotten so big". My mom responded she did not know in a bewildered voice. It hurt me because I felt that I had let her down. I was young and all I wanted was my family's approval. I wanted to make my mother proud, and to set a good example for my little sister. I believed that if I became thin, that I would accomplish both of these goals. And determined as I was, I did it: I ate grapefruit, drank water, and run consistently. I ran around the outside of our house several times, five times a day for the entire 100 day summer. Success! Everyone would be so proud... Or so I thought.

I lost so much weight between sixth and seventh grade that people thought I had an eating disorder! It hurt me that people thought I was anorexic. Once again, my weight was rearing up and taking over my life conversation. But I rationalized that it was better for everyone to believe I had an eating disorder than to once again be "the big girl".

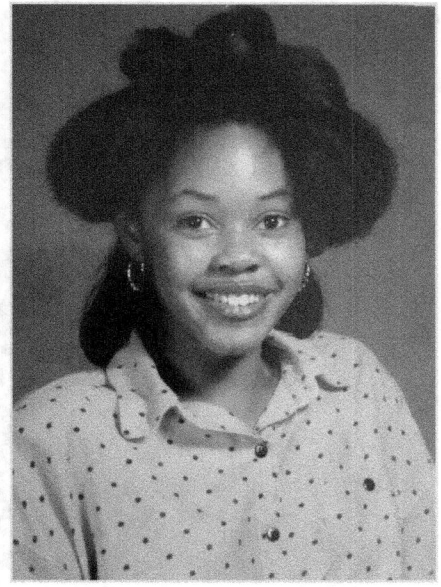

Me, seventh grade.
(I was rocking that shirt and my hair was oh-so-fly!

To maintain my weight, I started giving up things I loved. I had given up pork by the eighth grade. But because my weight loss methods were not life style changes consistent with healthy body image and self love, I could not maintain it. When I went off to college, I picked up the Freshman 15. My answer to this seeming catastrophe: I became a gym rat. I ran, took cardio classes, and lifted weights almost seven days a week. But I must have known subconsciously that something else would be required to maintain weight loss because I also began reading labels on the foods I ate.

I decided that fat was bad - all fat - so I once again gave up something I loved: cube steak. I remember one night making a cube steak in my dorm (totally against regulations, so don't tell). It was delicious! But a couple of hours after eating it, I got sick, and decided: no fat for me. I got down to a size six and continued to scrutinize food labels. I was determined to eliminate that awful, nasty fat from life!

After graduation, I befriended a co-worker who was also a fitness instructor. She guided me through a period of extraordinary balance in my life (compared to what I had been doing) where I ate small meals every day and allowed myself one "cheat day" each week. It worked well... until I got married and the extra pounds came back.

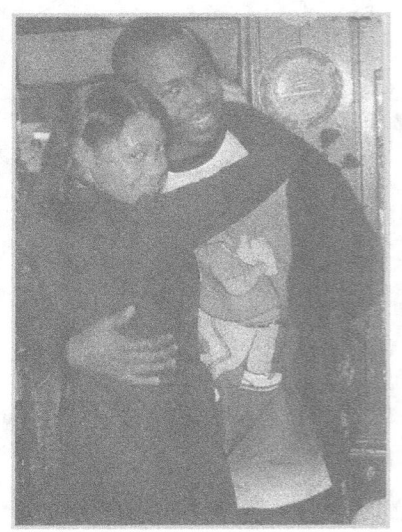

You know by now that I was not going to take this lying down, so I turned to various diets, supplements, and cleanses. I lost the weight and was thin, but it required incredible focus and a lot of effort. At the time, I did not mind,

With my hubby, newlywed bliss.

since I was performing - I was an actress, and it was necessary to maintain my weight. My perspective of healthy was cereal bars and anything that had a "healthy" label or endorsement. It never crossed my mind that the government would allow companies to make claims they knew to be false and/or misleading...

Me, *holding up REAL healthy foods and snacks.*

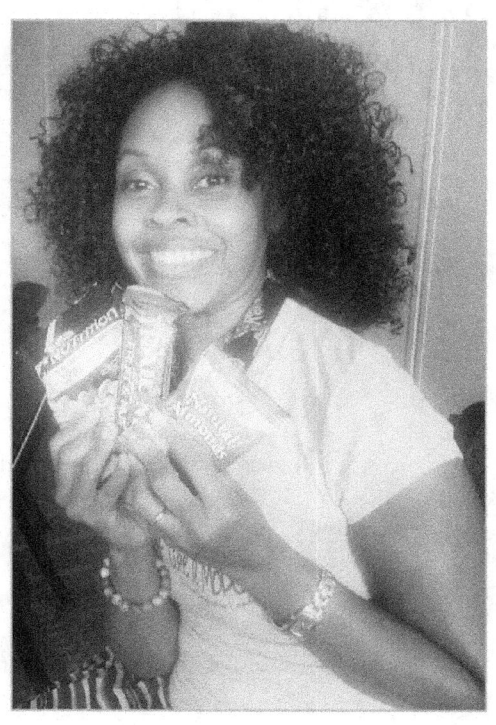

Once I realized that every label was not to be trusted, I began exploring other ways to maintain my weight. I eventually fell into the vegetarian lifestyle. I loved it, but when I became pregnant, things got a bit crazy. I craved meat with a vengeance, but could not eat it... along with a number of things. I was one of "those women" who lost weight the first trimester because I could not keep anything down, well, except my emotions.

I was on an emotional roller coaster! While I wanted children, we were not expecting them so soon in our marriage. I became depressed because I believed becoming a mother before I had achieved my career goals would be the monkey wrench to unhinge my grand life vision. I spent months searching for female mentors who were fulfilling their dreams with families, women who could serve as guides and support for me. After a while, I had an epiphany: I could be my own guide, chart my own way! Look what I had done so far in my life - why would that need to stop?

So I "got my mind right" and pressed on to have a really good pregnancy. My biggest problem? Eating enough! Ha, what a change embracing my current circumstances made. I had come full circle - from the girl who ate too much and was hefty to the woman who ate too little and deemed anorexic to now the soon-to-be-mom who did not care and was eating to provide her baby the recommended amount of protein.

I still did not eat meat, so I turned to soy. It was the new health rage, and was loaded with protein. But temptation reared its ugly head. One night I was sitting on the couch and my husband had a chicken mini from KFC. It smelled so good! I debated internally and finally asked for a "taste" which lead to me eating the entire mini and that concluded my almost year of vegetarianism.

After birth, breast feeding took care of my pregnancy weight and I became a "part time vegetarian": I still stayed away from beef and pork, but ate meat every other month. (I was a flexitarian before it was defined.)

After my second child about three years later, I found myself smaller than I had ever been in my life: a size 2. Woo-hoo, a 2?! Who would have thought the elementary kid that was wearing misses, the 120 pound kid, would ever see a two. I accepted it like a badge of honor. However, a holistic co-worker, who was also an iridologist, told me that I was underweight. I quickly dismissed her statement as inconsequential. I was determined to ride the "thin train" as long as I could, and I did for several years.

The stress of modern day life led to me gaining a few pounds, so I got up to a size four, and I held steady for quite some time. I realized that if I wanted to maintain for good that I would need to consume more nutrients, and do so without consuming more food.

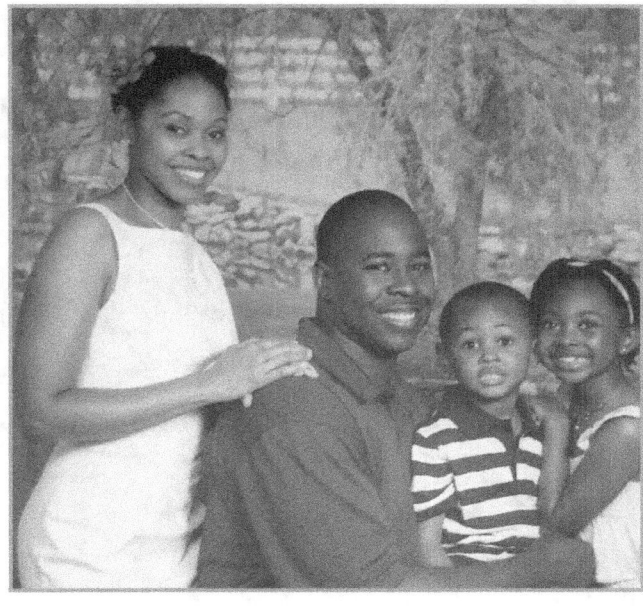

Me with my wonderful family (Picture taken about the time I realized I needed more nutrients.)

I compared the quality of things I had eaten in the past with my new cravings and realized that my old eating habits were depleting me of energy instead of giving it to me. So I became "gangsta" about my food, totally focused on eating only things that were good for me. And I determined that I would be the final judge as to what was healthy and what was not - I stopped relying on labels and claims that clearly did not amount to much.

This is about the time that I began to delve deeper into the green smoothie world. This was the key to maintaining a sense of balance with my weight struggle. Even though I had been "small" for several years, I still harbored the fear that I would become overweight again and subjected to the scorn from childhood that still resided in my heart. But I need not have worried - help was on the way!

After I had sold my family and close friends on the green smoothies, I began to really began to line up all aspects of my life. I was exercising about four times a week, eating food from the local Farmer's Market, and volunteering in the community to contribute my talents to the world.

I was on a roll! I had mastered "it" - my health, my fears, my struggles! I discovered the unique formula for MY optimal health. I now knew how to be an active individual with just enough exercise. I held steady at a size four, and it was at this place that I realized that size does not equal health. Yes, this nation has an obesity epidemic and there are many issues concerning that. But smaller does not all times mean healthier.

It's funny: after spending so much time worrying about my weight, it never occurred to me there would be something else out there that would take me down an even darker and twistier path...

5 MY PERSONAL TIPPING POINT - PART 2

I began this book recounting my encounter with a longtime friend Chantae. There is another part of the story that I am just now becoming comfortable sharing with the world after several years of hiding...

After I shared with Chantae my "secret" to maintaining weight loss, the conversation went into a direction that was unavoidable. "I like your head wrap," she stated. "You can pull that off, you have the face for it."

A casual passerby might have thought Chantae was simply letting me know that I could take off my head wrap in light of the heat, but she and I knew better. "It" was a kind way of saying "bald".

I calmly replied, "I saw you liked the picture." I had posted a picture on Facebook about a week prior in honor of Alopecia month displaying my bald head. I honestly can't remember if she asked directly, but I took a deep breath and bravely shared my story.

It was the summer of 2012, and I was a health coach. I had tried almost every diet or eating style under the sun, so I was quite knowledgeable in this area and could give my clients recommendations based on experience. I felt my thighs becoming jiggly so I began working with a personal trainer, and I also wanted to connect to help others with their eating. I was finding my tribe. I was eating more plant based foods, exercising, and enjoying life trying to build my business. One day I noticed a tiny bald spot on my nape. Not really concerned too much, I thought maybe it was too much tension because of the hairstyle I usually wear. After a couple of months I noticed it hadn't gotten better so I made a doctor's appointment. Unfortunately for me appointments would not be available for about 4 months, so I waited.

The doctor had no clue what could be causing the baldness, and referred me to a dermatologist - that took another 4 months. During my waiting period, the dermatologist suggested that I document my journey through pictures. I did, and the hair loss became ten times worse: that small spot was now a huge patch that went from the nape of my neck, up the back of my head, and circled around my ears. When I finally got in to the dermatologist, she diagnosed me with Alopecia. We tried shots and cream to stimulate re-growth, but after three months, nothing.

My dermatologist then confessed that in cases - like mine - it usually doesn't grow back. I was flummoxed. After almost a year, NOW you tell me that my hair is not going to grow back?!

Although not completely defeated, I was bummed out. My family and friends to the rescue! After talking it through and much prayer, I began to seek out holistic options. After my struggles with weight and acceptance, I believed that I could find a natural food and/or herb based solution to heal me. Combined with eating right, taking my recommended vitamins and supplements, I believed - and still believe - that all things are possible.

I returned to my doctor for a full set of tests, and she said my labs looked perfect. I did a ton of research and found a naturopath not too far from where I lived. We worked diligently for quite some time, but I did not experience any re-growth. I tried to remain positive, but by this time I began to feel as if I was cursed. Here I was, a health coach, with health degrees, and I now had a health concern such as this. Each time I looked into the mirror I saw a failure. How could I have allowed this to happen?

In an effort to bring more positive feelings towards myself, and reclaim a sense of control of my destiny, I took a pair of clippers and cut my hair low - like "in the Army now" low. It's so ironic that at the time of my "imbalance" I was developing a concept to start a hair blog. For as long as I can remember, I had received compliments about my hair - the color, strength, thickness, length - everything. I wanted to create a community for women to share their hair stories, even though for me, hair had never been a big issue - I respected it, and liked the way it looked, but I did not spend a lot of time obsessing over it. But now... now that it is gone, without any explanation as to how or why, was - and still is - hard to accept.

[*My transformation.*]

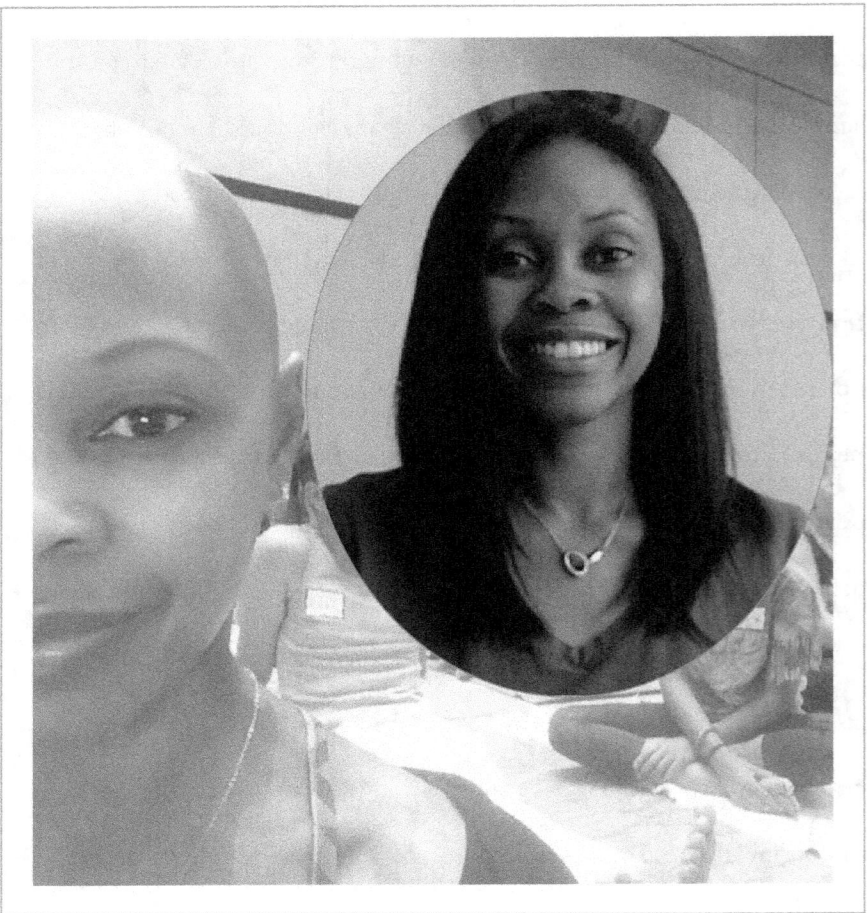

A year later, we relocated to a larger city and my hair began to thrive. I resumed my search for a naturopathic doctor and found one I really liked.

The problem - the pills! We began a supplement regimen to support all the bodily systems. I was literally taking 13 pills a day - I had a pill box! I was so frustrated: I was doing the very thing I did not want to do in my elderly years - taking a butt load of pills. Nevertheless, I continued to take the pills, as I believed my body could heal with the proper support.

Well, while taking these pills, I noticed that my hips were spreading. I had become very sedentary. I was exercising less and eating with more abandon due to the start of my Master's degree course work. I really did not have any more time in my day to add activities, so I decided to modify my diet. I decided to do a high fat, low carb diet to rev up my metabolism. After seeing a nutritionist, I realized several micronutrients were missing from my diet, and some were the same as those that contribute to hair loss. I began to eat more fermented foods to support my gut, and took iron supplements for hair and nails support. Then it happened: the front of my hairline began to fade. I saw it, but I tried to stay calm - this had happened before, it would grow back. I told myself not to stress, to just keep an eye on it and meditate more. But then my edges and the front of my hairline disappeared to the point where I could no longer camouflage my hair loss. There was no more hair to leave out for my lace front wigs, no more hair to smooth over my half-wigs (or falls). I began to wear full wigs because without my hair, I felt I looked sick.

I had become unrecognizable to myself.

So I did the one thing I could do to take total control of the situation - I shaved it off. All off. I reclaimed my power, my sense of control. And I like it. It's funky, it's edgy, and it's chique. I dress my bald head up with large rimmed glasses, statement jewelry, popping make up, and sometimes head wraps.

Sometimes I fall into despair about my hair, but the days are becoming fewer and further between. I have not given up on being healed, but I am learning to accept my "in the meantime" experience.

[*My choice.*]

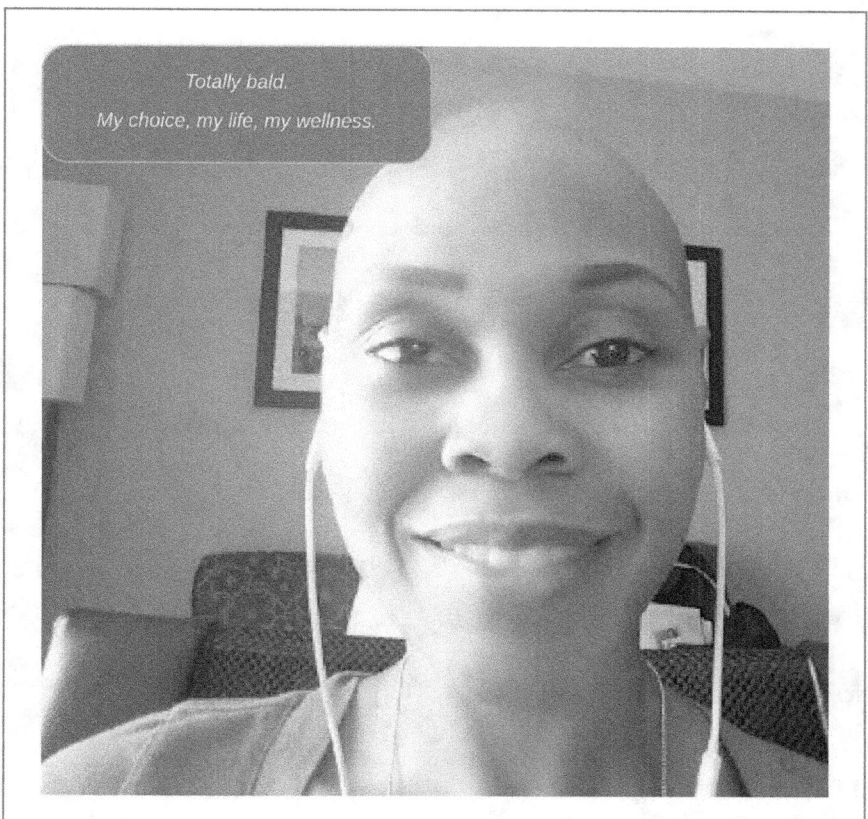

6 CONCLUSION

Today, I am in my late thirties, and weigh 125 pounds. At five feet, three inches, I look pretty good. I could probably tighten up a bit, but I look and feel good.

I eat what is considered better than the standard American diet (SAD) - most days. And I am slowly coming to accept that I have an auto-immune condition that causes Alopecia. There is so little research on the condition because it is considered cosmetic in nature and most doctors don't take it seriously (I actually had one say to me, "Oh, it's just hair loss").

So how do I, the health coach, the woman who preaches balance and variety, end up with nutritional deficiencies (iron and vitamin D) and hair loss? Genes. Yes, there are just some things that we are more susceptible to experience. It does not mean we have to take it lying down and not try to find ways to correct it. It just means that it will take some creativity and will power to overcome our DNA.

I say all of this to leave with you this statement: health and wellness are a journey, not a battle. A journey is a long trip, and there are experiences that are had along the way. A battle is a skirmish, to be fought and won - and is over rather succinctly. Your health and wellness state are life-long experiences unique to you. And when you find something on that journey that helps you feel better, embrace it. For me, it is the Green Smoothie. I am better when I have my smoothie – sometimes in the morning, midday, or even late night. There is no specific time or even formula. But this is how I got started and why I remain committed.

Throughout my journey I have found and still discovering that when I don't make the best health choices for my body – food, mindset, spiritual, and physical- there is a direct impact on my life. Health, wellness, and nutrition are so much more than what we consume, but food is a major factor and great place to start.

Interested in the "Number Two" Thing You Can Do For Your Health?

Schedule a free health consultation with a health coach who can help you sift through all the variables that are unique to you. There is absolutely no obligation, but you'll walk away from the session with greater clarity about the unique lifestyle and nutrition habits you'll need to get yourself on your way to a truly healthy, happy life. Contact me today!

To your health!

ABOUT THE AUTHOR

Nasha Shandri, CHC, LMT

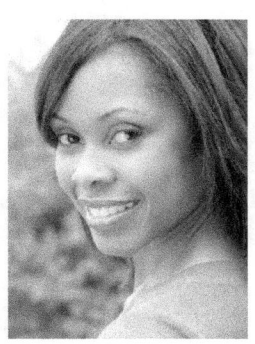 Nasha is a holistic health coach that has received training in over 100 dietary theories. She also a certified massage therapist and professional speaker, and completing her Master of Science degree as a functional integrative clinical nutritionist. Nasha combines her education and industry experience to develop programs with her clients to achieve their goals. Over the years she has found that there is no lack of programs and coaches to help people lose weight; but few are able to support how to maintain the weight loss. Her personal journey has created a sacred space of compassion when partnering with clients. She is living her journey – assisting clients to live theirs. Her passion is supporting unstoppable men and women in creating harmony between nutrition and lifestyle. "I assist road warriors, professionals, and homepreneurs maintain their weight and release stress to become healthy, vibrant, experts of their bodies. My approach is practical only if you have decided your health is no longer an option. I look forward to helping you get across the bridge of conception to the reality of healthy living. You can experience nutrition and lifestyle synergy."

Disclaimer: this book if for informational purposes only. Please consult your physician before making any major dietary changes.